MW01289949

This Book Belongs To:

. . . .

. . . .

. . . .

TypeOneToddler.com

Emergency Contacts

Type One Toddler

Shot Location

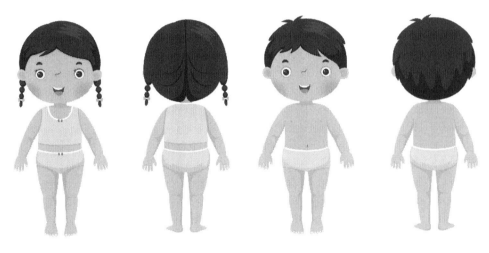

Notes

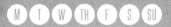

	Time	Blood Sugar	Carbs	Insulin	Notes
Breakfast					
Snack					
Lunch					
Snack					
Dinner					
Bedtime					
Night					

Shot Location

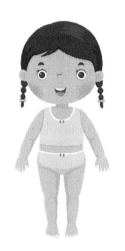 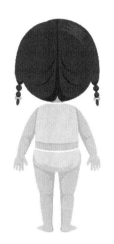 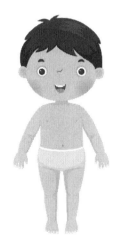 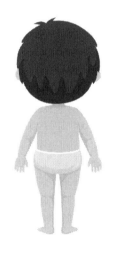

Notes

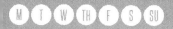
	Time	Blood Sugar	Carbs	Insulin	Notes
Breakfast					
Snack					
Lunch					
Snack					
Dinner					
Bedtime					
Night					

Shot Location

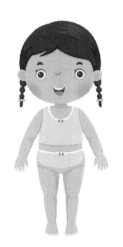 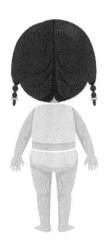 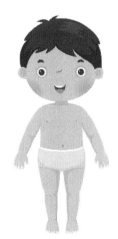 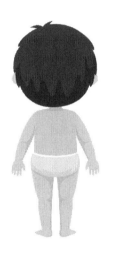

Notes

	Time	Blood Sugar	Carbs	Insulin	Notes
Breakfast					
Snack					
Lunch					
Snack					
Dinner					
Bedtime					
Night					

Shot Location

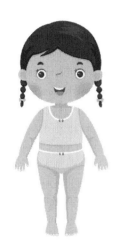 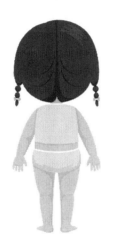 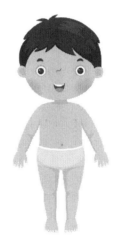 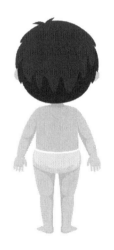

Notes

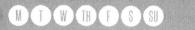
	Time	Blood Sugar	Carbs	Insulin	Notes
Breakfast					
Snack					
Lunch					
Snack					
Dinner					
Bedtime					
Night					

Shot Location

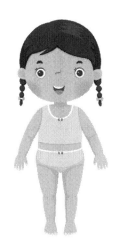 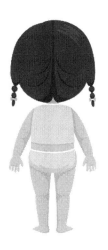 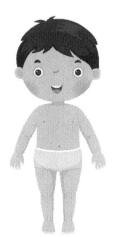 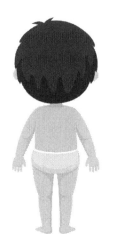

Notes

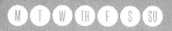
	Time	Blood Sugar	Carbs	Insulin	Notes
Breakfast					
Snack					
Lunch					
Snack					
Dinner					
Bedtime					
Night					

Shot Location

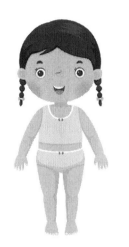 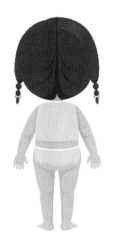 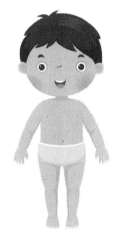 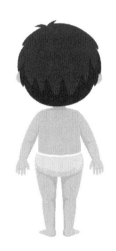

Notes

	Time	Blood Sugar	Carbs	Insulin	Notes
Breakfast					
Snack					
Lunch					
Snack					
Dinner					
Bedtime					
Night					

Shot Location

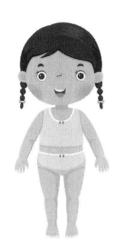 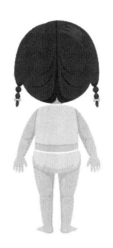 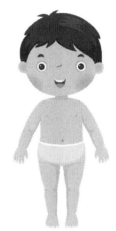 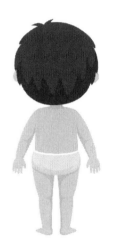

Notes

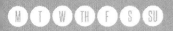
	Time	Blood Sugar	Carbs	Insulin	Notes
Breakfast					
Snack					
Lunch					
Snack					
Dinner					
Bedtime					
Night					

Shot Location

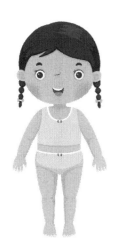 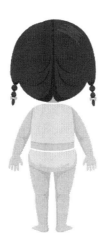 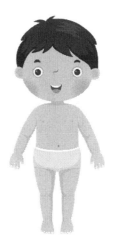 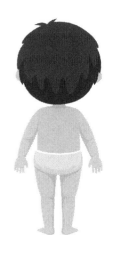

Notes

	Time	Blood Sugar	Carbs	Insulin	Notes
Breakfast					
Snack					
Lunch					
Snack					
Dinner					
Bedtime					
Night					

Shot Location

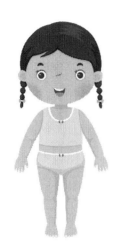 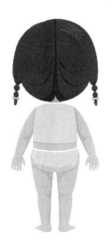 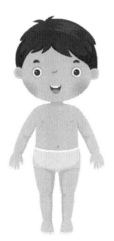 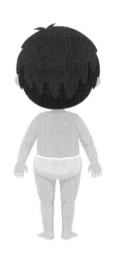

Notes

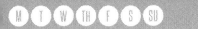
	Time	Blood Sugar	Carbs	Insulin	Notes
Breakfast					
Snack					
Lunch					
Snack					
Dinner					
Bedtime					
Night					

Shot Location

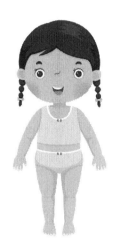 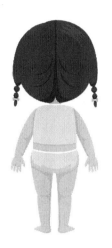 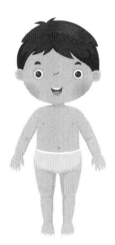 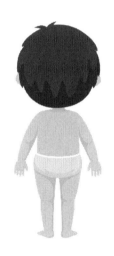

Notes

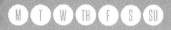

	Time	Blood Sugar	Carbs	Insulin	Notes
Breakfast					
Snack					
Lunch					
Snack					
Dinner					
Bedtime					
Night					

Shot Location

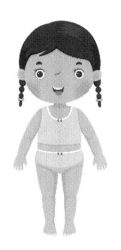 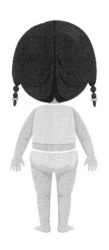 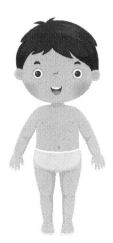 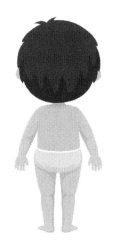

Notes

	Time	Blood Sugar	Carbs	Insulin	Notes
Breakfast					
Snack					
Lunch					
Snack					
Dinner					
Bedtime					
Night					

Shot Location

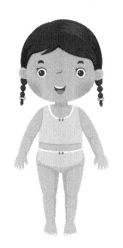 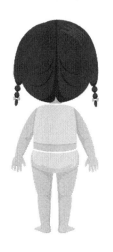 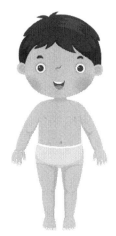 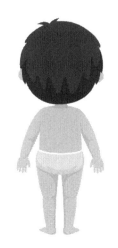

Notes

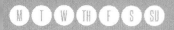
	Time	Blood Sugar	Carbs	Insulin	Notes
Breakfast					
Snack					
Lunch					
Snack					
Dinner					
Bedtime					
Night					

Shot Location

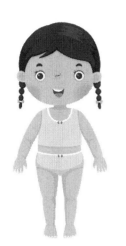 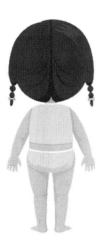 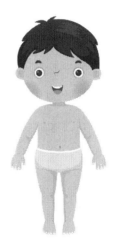 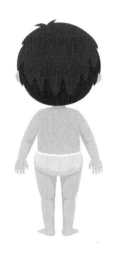

Notes

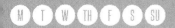
	Time	Blood Sugar	Carbs	Insulin	Notes
Breakfast					
Snack					
Lunch					
Snack					
Dinner					
Bedtime					
Night					

Shot Location

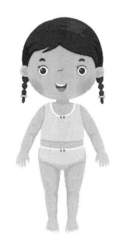 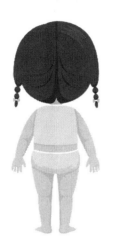 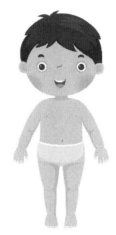 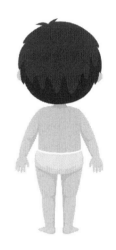

Notes

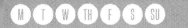
	Time	Blood Sugar	Carbs	Insulin	Notes
Breakfast					
Snack					
Lunch					
Snack					
Dinner					
Bedtime					
Night					

Shot Location

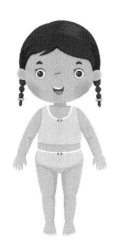 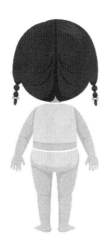 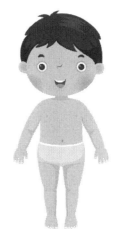 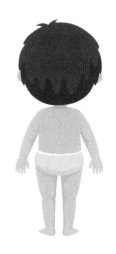

Notes

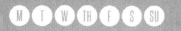

T W TH F S SU

Date: /   /

	Time	Blood Sugar	Carbs	Insulin	Notes
Breakfast					
Snack					
Lunch					
Snack					
Dinner					
Bedtime					
Night					

Shot Location

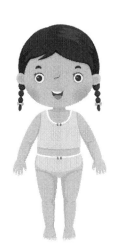 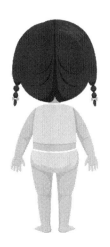 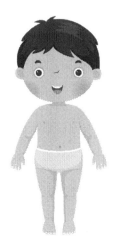 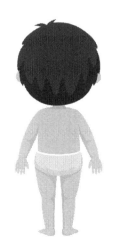

Notes

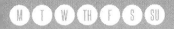
	Time	Blood Sugar	Carbs	Insulin	Notes
Breakfast					
Snack					
Lunch					
Snack					
Dinner					
Bedtime					
Night					

Shot Location

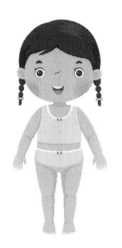 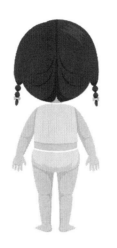 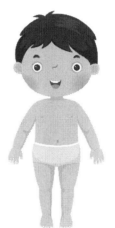 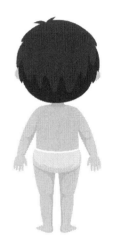

Notes

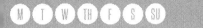
	Time	Blood Sugar	Carbs	Insulin	Notes
Breakfast					
Snack					
Lunch					
Snack					
Dinner					
Bedtime					
Night					

Shot Location

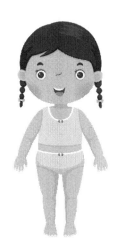 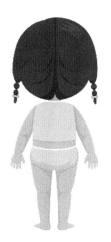 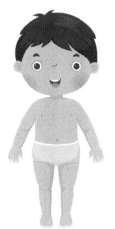 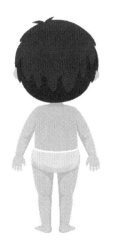

Notes

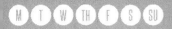
	Time	Blood Sugar	Carbs	Insulin	Notes
Breakfast					
Snack					
Lunch					
Snack					
Dinner					
Bedtime					
Night					

Shot Location

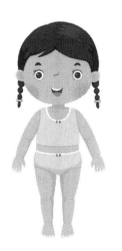 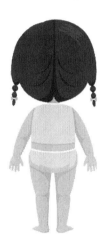 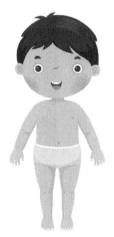 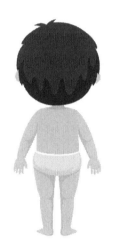

Notes

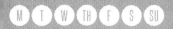
	Time	Blood Sugar	Carbs	Insulin	Notes
Breakfast					
Snack					
Lunch					
Snack					
Dinner					
Bedtime					
Night					

Shot Location

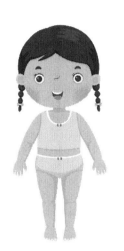 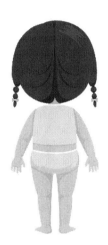 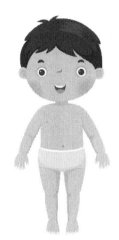 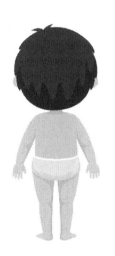

Notes

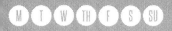

	Time	Blood Sugar	Carbs	Insulin	Notes
Breakfast					
Snack					
Lunch					
Snack					
Dinner					
Bedtime					
Night					

Shot Location

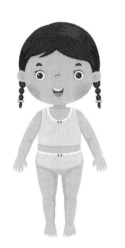 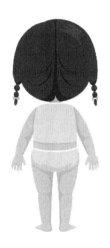 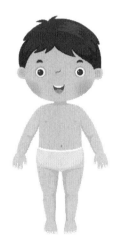 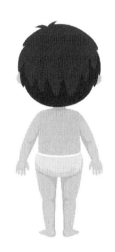

Notes

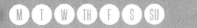
	Time	Blood Sugar	Carbs	Insulin	Notes
Breakfast					
Snack					
Lunch					
Snack					
Dinner					
Bedtime					
Night					

Shot Location

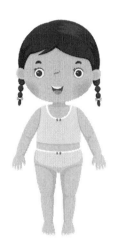 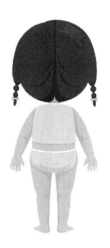 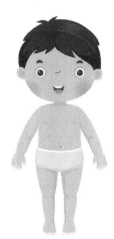 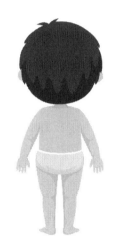

Notes

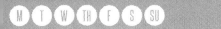
	Time	Blood Sugar	Carbs	Insulin	Notes
Breakfast					
Snack					
Lunch					
Snack					
Dinner					
Bedtime					
Night					

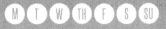
Shot Location

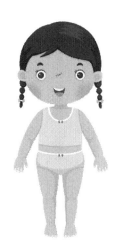 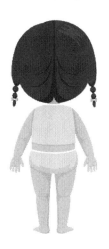 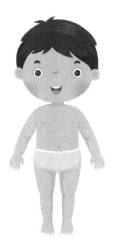 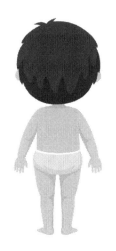

Notes

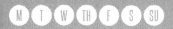
	Time	Blood Sugar	Carbs	Insulin	Notes
Breakfast					
Snack					
Lunch					
Snack					
Dinner					
Bedtime					
Night					

Shot Location

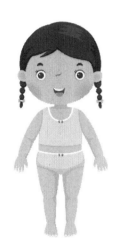 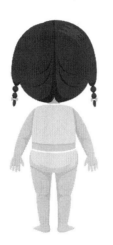 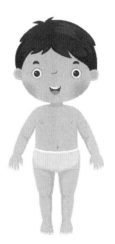 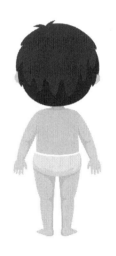

Notes

	Time	Blood Sugar	Carbs	Insulin	Notes
Breakfast					
Snack					
Lunch					
Snack					
Dinner					
Bedtime					
Night					

Shot Location

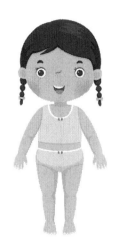 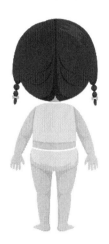 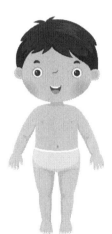 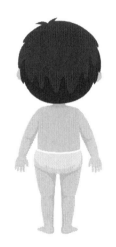

Notes

	Time	Blood Sugar	Carbs	Insulin	Notes
Breakfast					
Snack					
Lunch					
Snack					
Dinner					
Bedtime					
Night					

Shot Location

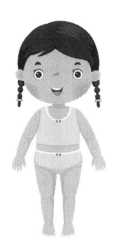 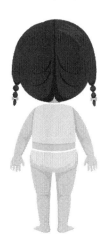 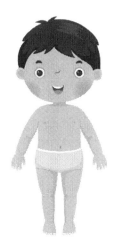 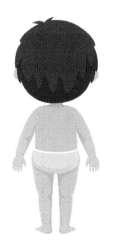

Notes

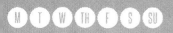

	Time	Blood Sugar	Carbs	Insulin	Notes
Breakfast					
Snack					
Lunch					
Snack					
Dinner					
Bedtime					
Night					

Shot Location

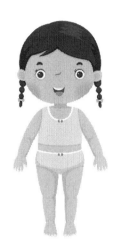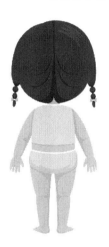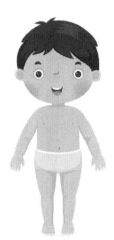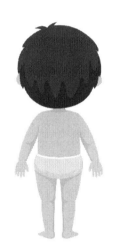

Notes

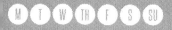
	Time	Blood Sugar	Carbs	Insulin	Notes
Breakfast					
Snack					
Lunch					
Snack					
Dinner					
Bedtime					
Night					

Shot Location

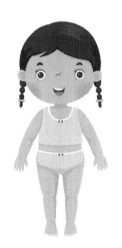 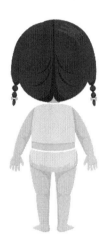 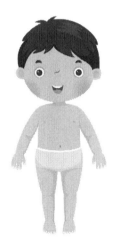 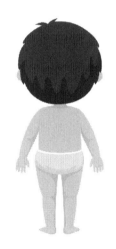

Notes

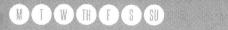

	Time	Blood Sugar	Carbs	Insulin	Notes
Breakfast					
Snack					
Lunch					
Snack					
Dinner					
Bedtime					
Night					

Shot Location

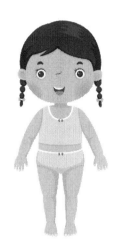 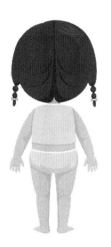 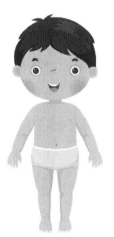 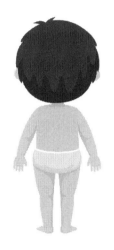

Notes

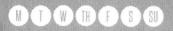
	Time	Blood Sugar	Carbs	Insulin	Notes
Breakfast					
Snack					
Lunch					
Snack					
Dinner					
Bedtime					
Night					

Shot Location

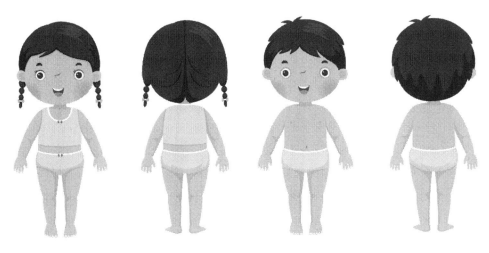

Notes

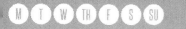
	Time	Blood Sugar	Carbs	Insulin	Notes
Breakfast					
Snack					
Lunch					
Snack					
Dinner					
Bedtime					
Night					

Shot Location

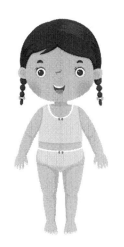 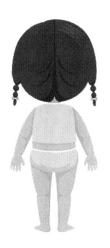 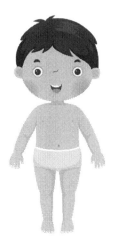 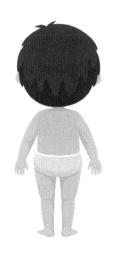

Notes

	Time	Blood Sugar	Carbs	Insulin	Notes
Breakfast					
Snack					
Lunch					
Snack					
Dinner					
Bedtime					
Night					

Shot Location

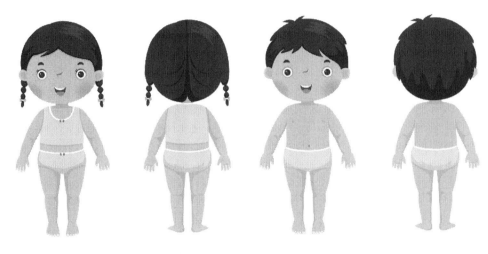

Notes

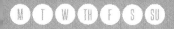
	Time	Blood Sugar	Carbs	Insulin	Notes
Breakfast					
Snack					
Lunch					
Snack					
Dinner					
Bedtime					
Night					

Shot Location

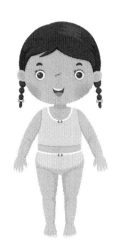 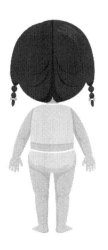 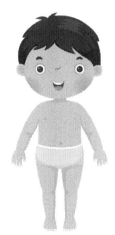 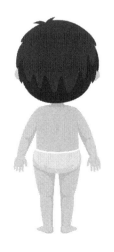

Notes

	Time	Blood Sugar	Carbs	Insulin	Notes
Breakfast					
Snack					
Lunch					
Snack					
Dinner					
Bedtime					
Night					

Shot Location

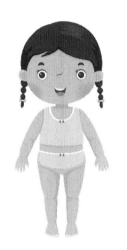 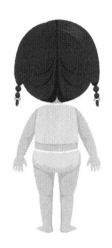 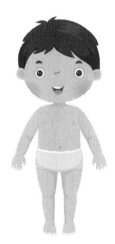 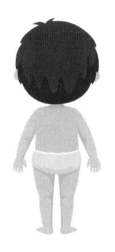

Notes

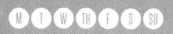
	Time	Blood Sugar	Carbs	Insulin	Notes
Breakfast					
Snack					
Lunch					
Snack					
Dinner					
Bedtime					
Night					

Shot Location

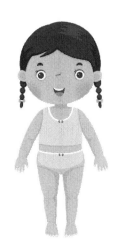 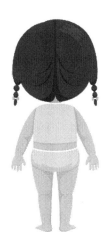 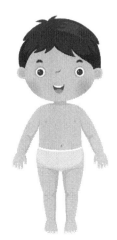 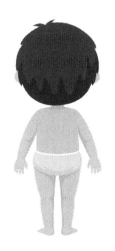

Notes

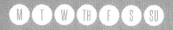
	Time	Blood Sugar	Carbs	Insulin	Notes
Breakfast					
Snack					
Lunch					
Snack					
Dinner					
Bedtime					
Night					

Shot Location

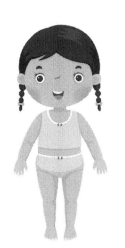 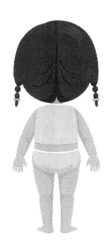 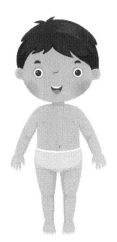 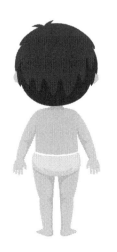

Notes

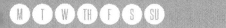

	Time	Blood Sugar	Carbs	Insulin	Notes
Breakfast					
Snack					
Lunch					
Snack					
Dinner					
Bedtime					
Night					

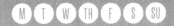
Shot Location

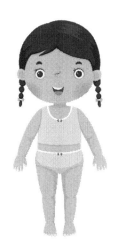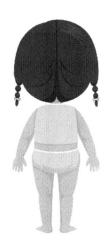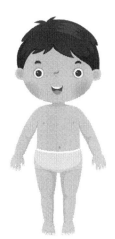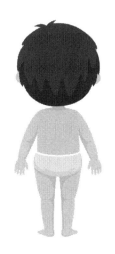

Notes

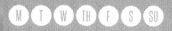

	Time	Blood Sugar	Carbs	Insulin	Notes
Breakfast					
Snack					
Lunch					
Snack					
Dinner					
Bedtime					
Night					

Shot Location

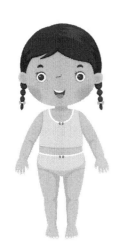 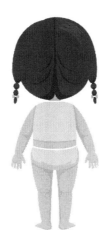 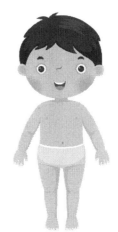 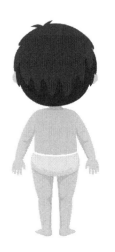

Notes

	Time	Blood Sugar	Carbs	Insulin	Notes
Breakfast					
Snack					
Lunch					
Snack					
Dinner					
Bedtime					
Night					

Shot Location

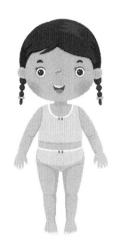 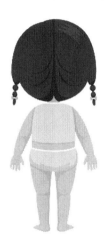 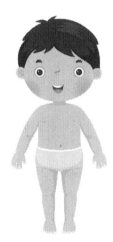 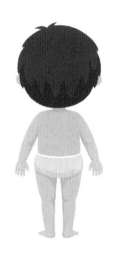

Notes

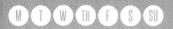
	Time	Blood Sugar	Carbs	Insulin	Notes
Breakfast					
Snack					
Lunch					
Snack					
Dinner					
Bedtime					
Night					

Shot Location

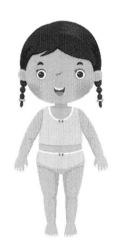 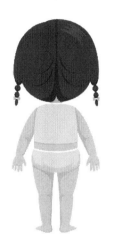 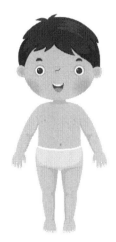 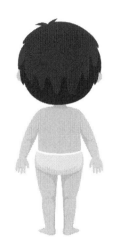

Notes

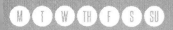
	Time	Blood Sugar	Carbs	Insulin	Notes
Breakfast					
Snack					
Lunch					
Snack					
Dinner					
Bedtime					
Night					

Shot Location

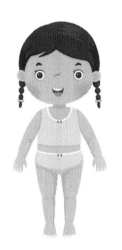 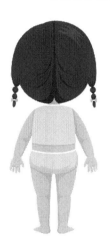 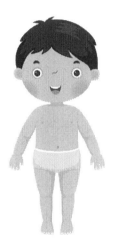 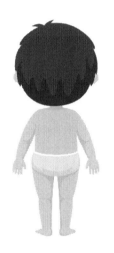

Notes

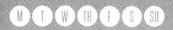
	Time	Blood Sugar	Carbs	Insulin	Notes
Breakfast					
Snack					
Lunch					
Snack					
Dinner					
Bedtime					
Night					

Shot Location

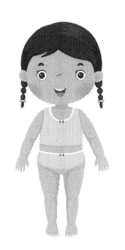 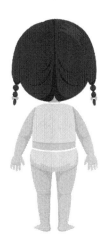 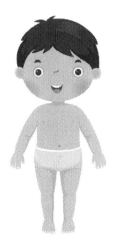 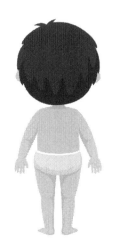

Notes

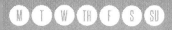
	Time	Blood Sugar	Carbs	Insulin	Notes
Breakfast					
Snack					
Lunch					
Snack					
Dinner					
Bedtime					
Night					

Shot Location

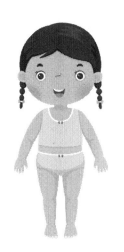 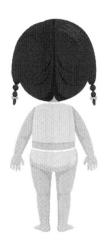 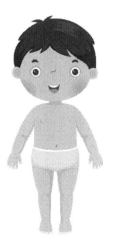 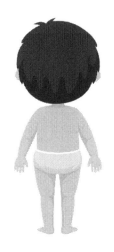

Notes

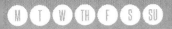
	Time	Blood Sugar	Carbs	Insulin	Notes
Breakfast					
Snack					
Lunch					
Snack					
Dinner					
Bedtime					
Night					

Shot Location

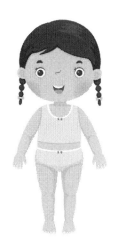 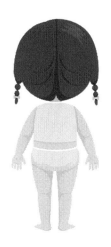 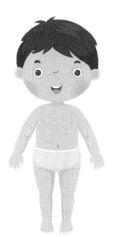 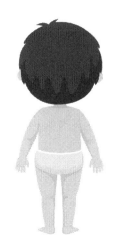

Notes

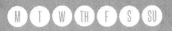
	Time	Blood Sugar	Carbs	Insulin	Notes
Breakfast					
Snack					
Lunch					
Snack					
Dinner					
Bedtime					
Night					

Shot Location

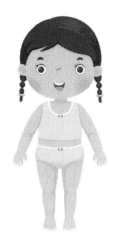 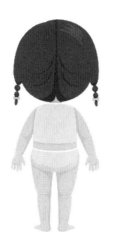 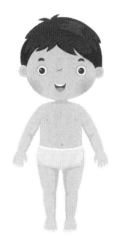 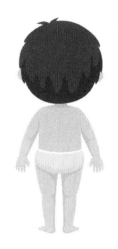

Notes

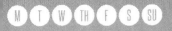

	Time	Blood Sugar	Carbs	Insulin	Notes
Breakfast					
Snack					
Lunch					
Snack					
Dinner					
Bedtime					
Night					

Shot Location

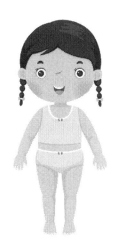 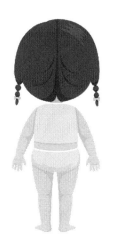 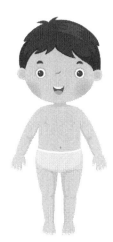 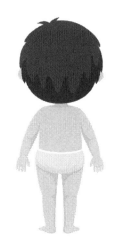

Notes

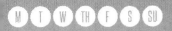
	Time	Blood Sugar	Carbs	Insulin	Notes
Breakfast					
Snack					
Lunch					
Snack					
Dinner					
Bedtime					
Night					

Shot Location

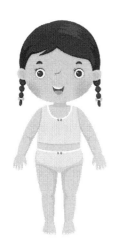 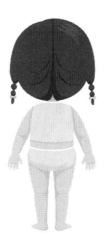 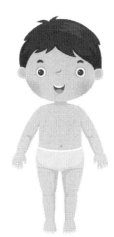 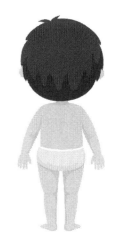

Notes

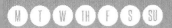

	Time	Blood Sugar	Carbs	Insulin	Notes
Breakfast					
Snack					
Lunch					
Snack					
Dinner					
Bedtime					
Night					

Shot Location

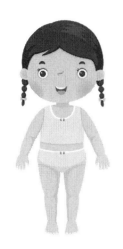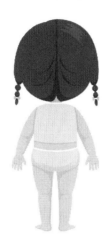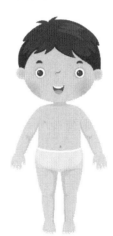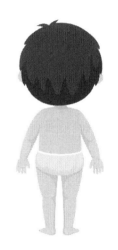

Notes

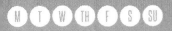
	Time	Blood Sugar	Carbs	Insulin	Notes
Breakfast					
Snack					
Lunch					
Snack					
Dinner					
Bedtime					
Night					

Shot Location

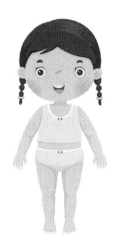 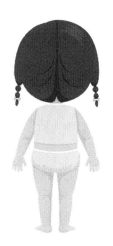 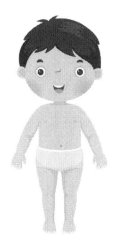 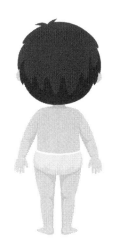

Notes

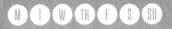
	Time	Blood Sugar	Carbs	Insulin	Notes
Breakfast					
Snack					
Lunch					
Snack					
Dinner					
Bedtime					
Night					

Shot Location

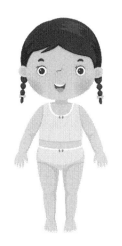 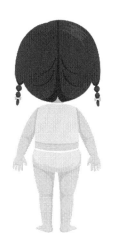 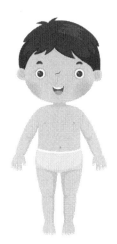 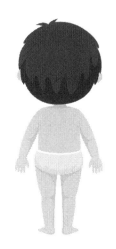

Notes

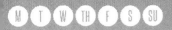
	Time	Blood Sugar	Carbs	Insulin	Notes
Breakfast					
Snack					
Lunch					
Snack					
Dinner					
Bedtime					
Night					

Shot Location

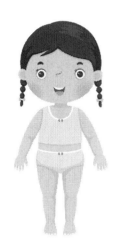 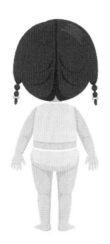 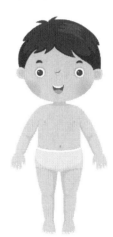 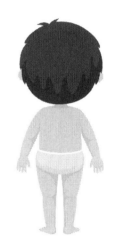

Notes

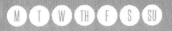
	Time	Blood Sugar	Carbs	Insulin	Notes
Breakfast					
Snack					
Lunch					
Snack					
Dinner					
Bedtime					
Night					

Shot Location

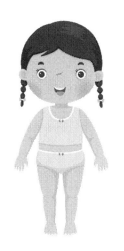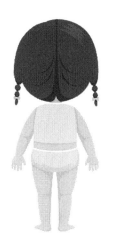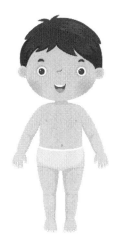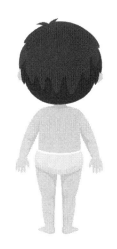

Notes

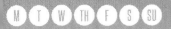
	Time	Blood Sugar	Carbs	Insulin	Notes
Breakfast					
Snack					
Lunch					
Snack					
Dinner					
Bedtime					
Night					

Shot Location

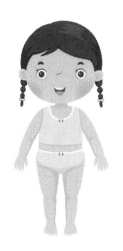 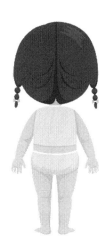 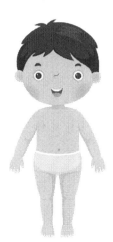 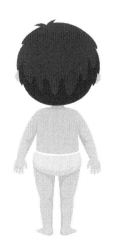

Notes

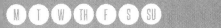 M T W TH F S SU

Date: / /

	Time	Blood Sugar	Carbs	Insulin	Notes
Breakfast					
Snack					
Lunch					
Snack					
Dinner					
Bedtime					
Night					

Shot Location

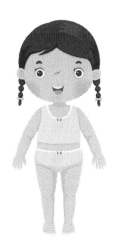 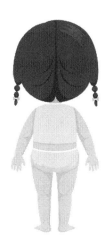 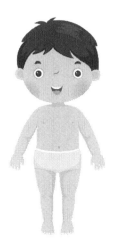 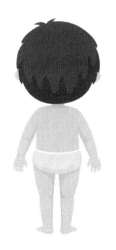

Notes

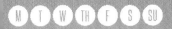
	Time	Blood Sugar	Carbs	Insulin	Notes
Breakfast					
Snack					
Lunch					
Snack					
Dinner					
Bedtime					
Night					

Shot Location

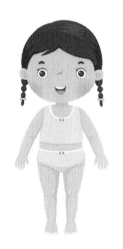 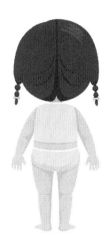 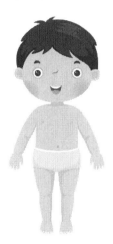 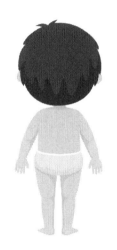

Notes

	Time	Blood Sugar	Carbs	Insulin	Notes
Breakfast					
Snack					
Lunch					
Snack					
Dinner					
Bedtime					
Night					

Shot Location

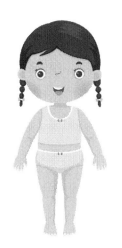 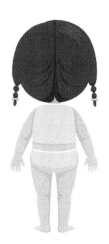 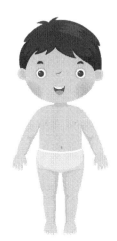 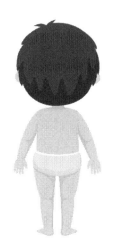

Notes

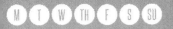
	Time	Blood Sugar	Carbs	Insulin	Notes
Breakfast					
Snack					
Lunch					
Snack					
Dinner					
Bedtime					
Night					

Shot Location

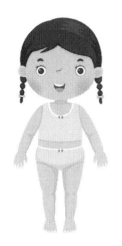 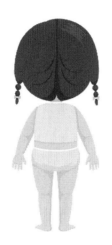 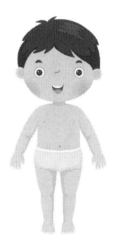 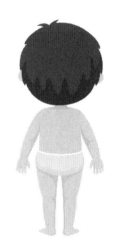

Notes

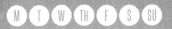
	Time	Blood Sugar	Carbs	Insulin	Notes
Breakfast					
Snack					
Lunch					
Snack					
Dinner					
Bedtime					
Night					

Shot Location

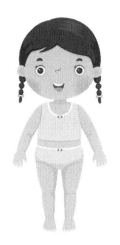 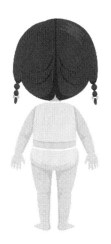 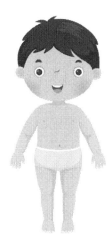 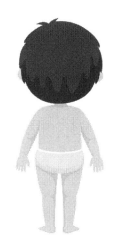

Notes

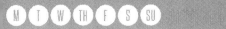
	Time	Blood Sugar	Carbs	Insulin	Notes
Breakfast					
Snack					
Lunch					
Snack					
Dinner					
Bedtime					
Night					

Shot Location

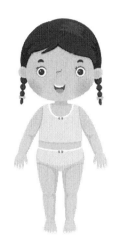 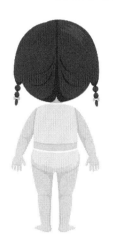 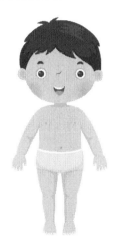 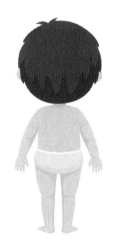

Notes

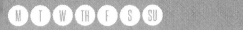
	Time	Blood Sugar	Carbs	Insulin	Notes
Breakfast					
Snack					
Lunch					
Snack					
Dinner					
Bedtime					
Night					

Shot Location

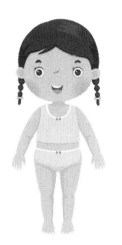 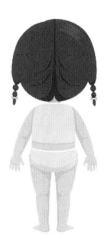 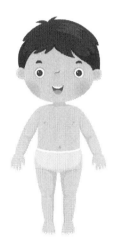 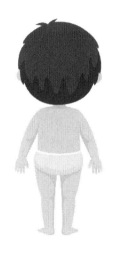

Notes

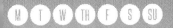
	Time	Blood Sugar	Carbs	Insulin	Notes
Breakfast					
Snack					
Lunch					
Snack					
Dinner					
Bedtime					
Night					

Shot Location

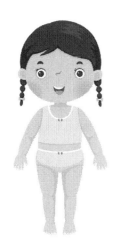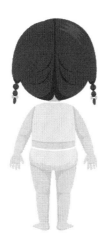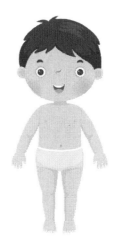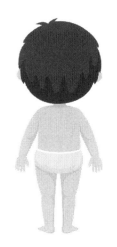

Notes

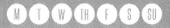

	Time	Blood Sugar	Carbs	Insulin	Notes
Breakfast					
Snack					
Lunch					
Snack					
Dinner					
Bedtime					
Night					

Shot Location

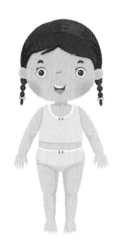 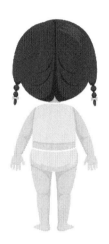 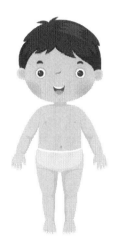 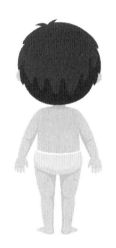

Notes

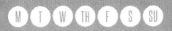
	Time	Blood Sugar	Carbs	Insulin	Notes
Breakfast					
Snack					
Lunch					
Snack					
Dinner					
Bedtime					
Night					

Shot Location

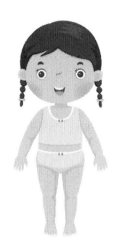 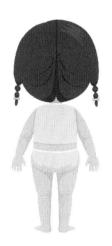 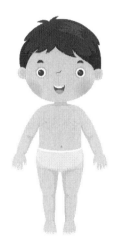 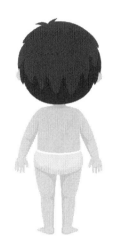

Notes

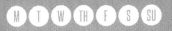

	Time	Blood Sugar	Carbs	Insulin	Notes
Breakfast					
Snack					
Lunch					
Snack					
Dinner					
Bedtime					
Night					

Shot Location

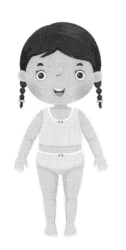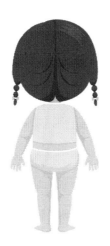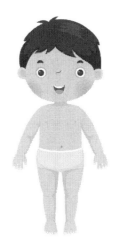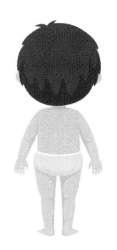

Notes

Date: / /

	Time	Blood Sugar	Carbs	Insulin	Notes
Breakfast					
Snack					
Lunch					
Snack					
Dinner					
Bedtime					
Night					

Shot Location

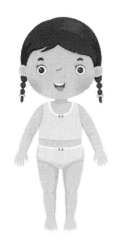 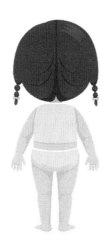 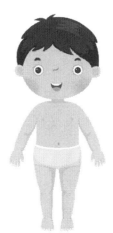 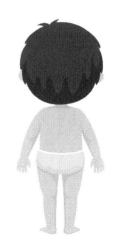

Notes

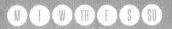
	Time	Blood Sugar	Carbs	Insulin	Notes
Breakfast					
Snack					
Lunch					
Snack					
Dinner					
Bedtime					
Night					

Shot Location

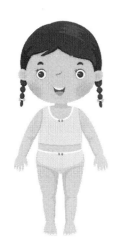 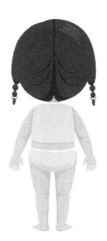 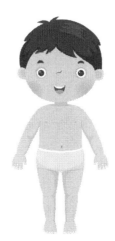 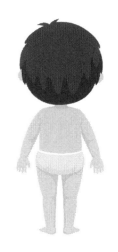

Notes

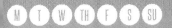
	Time	Blood Sugar	Carbs	Insulin	Notes
Breakfast					
Snack					
Lunch					
Snack					
Dinner					
Bedtime					
Night					

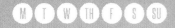
Shot Location

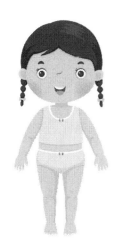 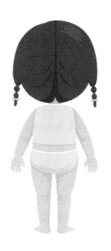 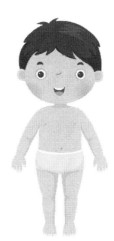 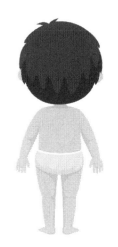

Notes

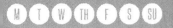

	Time	Blood Sugar	Carbs	Insulin	Notes
Breakfast					
Snack					
Lunch					
Snack					
Dinner					
Bedtime					
Night					

Shot Location

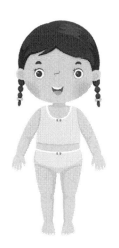 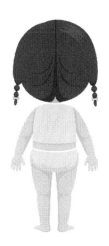 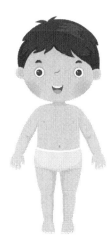 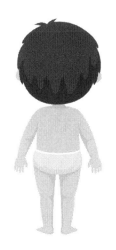

Notes

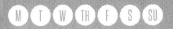

	Time	Blood Sugar	Carbs	Insulin	Notes
Breakfast					
Snack					
Lunch					
Snack					
Dinner					
Bedtime					
Night					

Shot Location

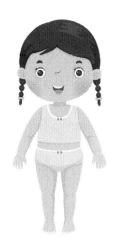 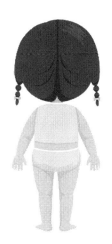 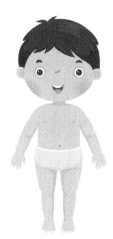 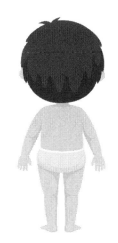

Notes

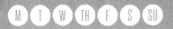
	Time	Blood Sugar	Carbs	Insulin	Notes
Breakfast					
Snack					
Lunch					
Snack					
Dinner					
Bedtime					
Night					

Shot Location

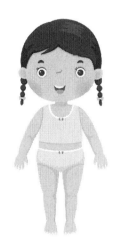 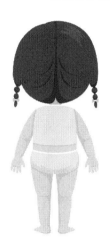 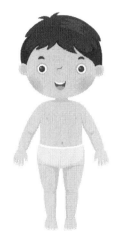 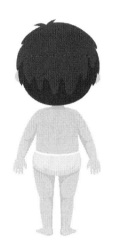

Notes

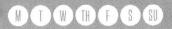
	Time	Blood Sugar	Carbs	Insulin	Notes
Breakfast					
Snack					
Lunch					
Snack					
Dinner					
Bedtime					
Night					

Shot Location

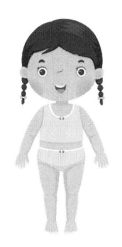 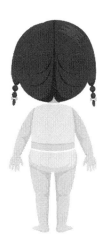 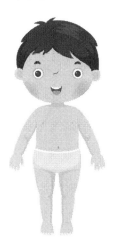 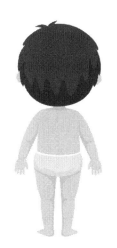

Notes

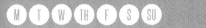
	Time	Blood Sugar	Carbs	Insulin	Notes
Breakfast					
Snack					
Lunch					
Snack					
Dinner					
Bedtime					
Night					

Shot Location

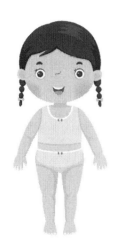 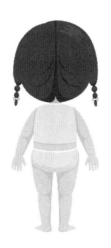 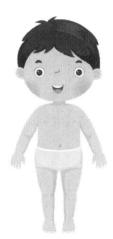 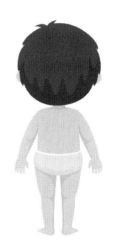

Notes

	Time	Blood Sugar	Carbs	Insulin	Notes
Breakfast					
Snack					
Lunch					
Snack					
Dinner					
Bedtime					
Night					

Shot Location

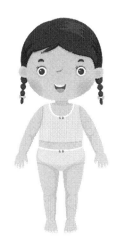 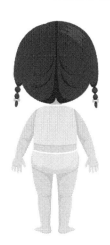 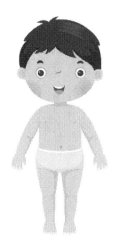 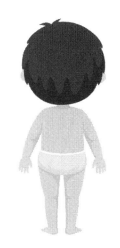

Notes

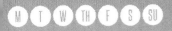
	Time	Blood Sugar	Carbs	Insulin	Notes
Breakfast					
Snack					
Lunch					
Snack					
Dinner					
Bedtime					
Night					

Shot Location

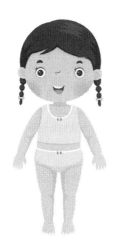 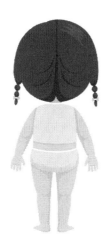 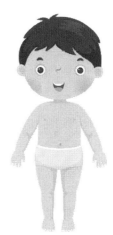 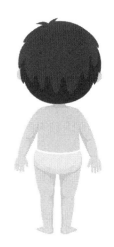

Notes

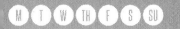

	Time	Blood Sugar	Carbs	Insulin	Notes
Breakfast					
Snack					
Lunch					
Snack					
Dinner					
Bedtime					
Night					

Shot Location

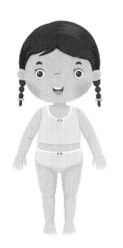 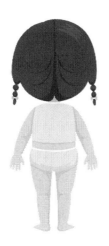 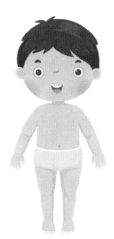 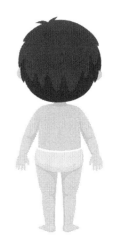

Notes

	Time	Blood Sugar	Carbs	Insulin	Notes
Breakfast					
Snack					
Lunch					
Snack					
Dinner					
Bedtime					
Night					

Shot Location

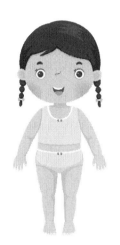 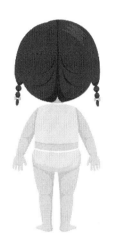 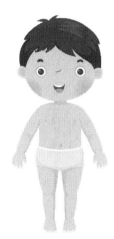 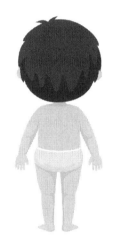

Notes

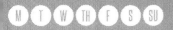
	Time	Blood Sugar	Carbs	Insulin	Notes
Breakfast					
Snack					
Lunch					
Snack					
Dinner					
Bedtime					
Night					

Shot Location

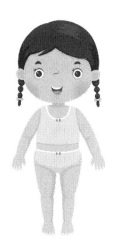 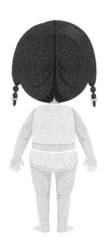 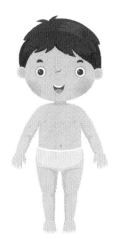 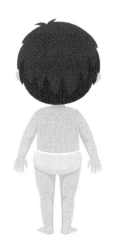

Notes

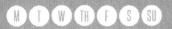
	Time	Blood Sugar	Carbs	Insulin	Notes
Breakfast					
Snack					
Lunch					
Snack					
Dinner					
Bedtime					
Night					

Shot Location

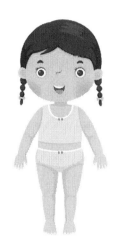 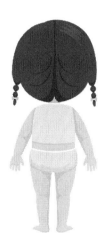 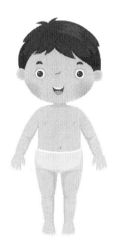 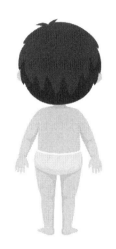

Notes

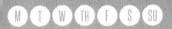

	Time	Blood Sugar	Carbs	Insulin	Notes
Breakfast					
Snack					
Lunch					
Snack					
Dinner					
Bedtime					
Night					

Shot Location

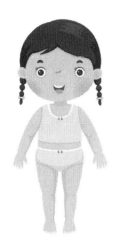 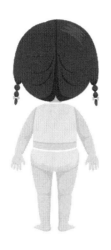 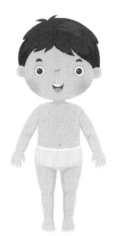 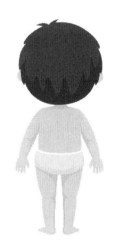

Notes

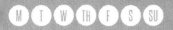
	Time	Blood Sugar	Carbs	Insulin	Notes
Breakfast					
Snack					
Lunch					
Snack					
Dinner					
Bedtime					
Night					

Shot Location

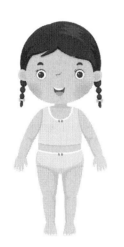 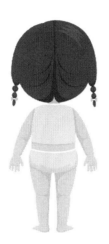 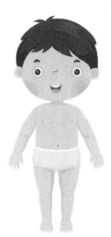 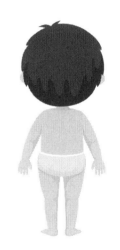

Notes

Date: / /

	Time	Blood Sugar	Carbs	Insulin	Notes
Breakfast					
Snack					
Lunch					
Snack					
Dinner					
Bedtime					
Night					

Shot Location

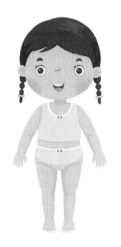 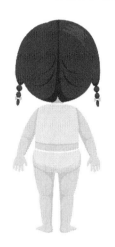 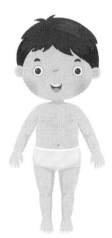 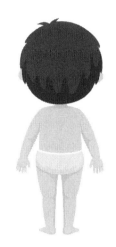

Notes

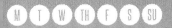
	Time	Blood Sugar	Carbs	Insulin	Notes
Breakfast					
Snack					
Lunch					
Snack					
Dinner					
Bedtime					
Night					

Shot Location

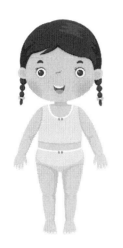 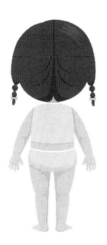 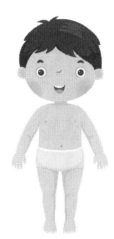 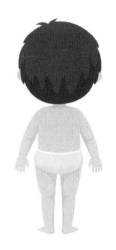

Notes

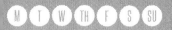
	Time	Blood Sugar	Carbs	Insulin	Notes
Breakfast					
Snack					
Lunch					
Snack					
Dinner					
Bedtime					
Night					

Shot Location

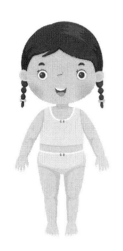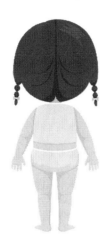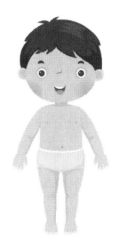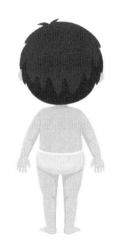

Notes

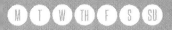
	Time	Blood Sugar	Carbs	Insulin	Notes
Breakfast					
Snack					
Lunch					
Snack					
Dinner					
Bedtime					
Night					

Shot Location

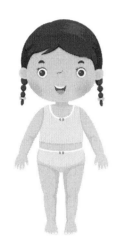 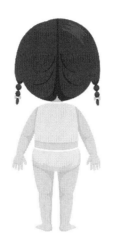 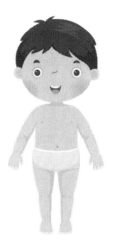 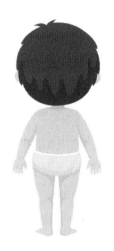

Notes

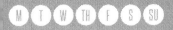
	Time	Blood Sugar	Carbs	Insulin	Notes
Breakfast					
Snack					
Lunch					
Snack					
Dinner					
Bedtime					
Night					

Type One Toddler

Made in the USA
Middletown, DE
27 April 2023

29530706R00097